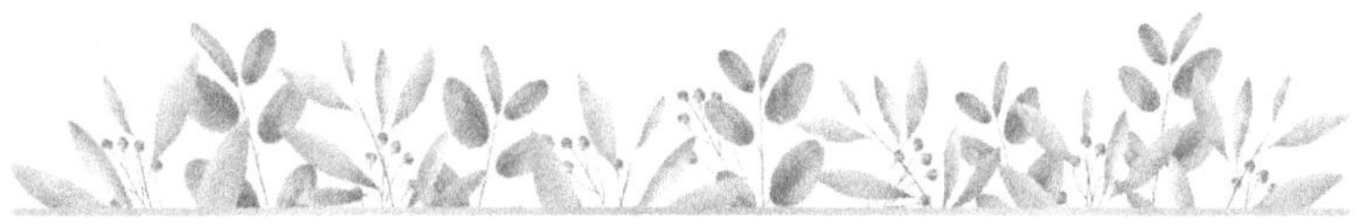

The Quick and Easy PCOS Diet Cookbook

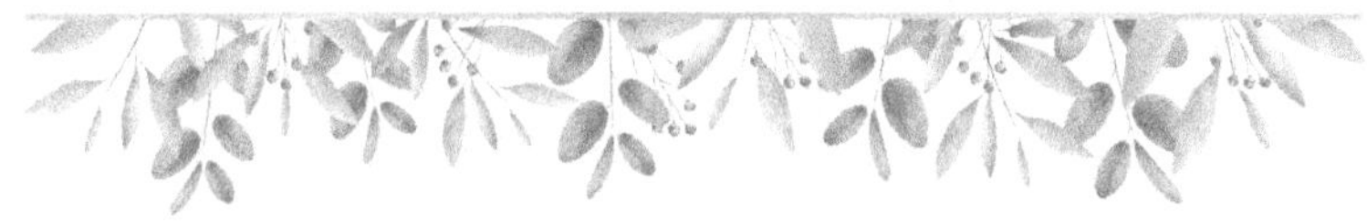

Nourishing Recipes for Hormone Balance, Insulin Resistance, Women's Health, Fertility, and More

Laura Zander

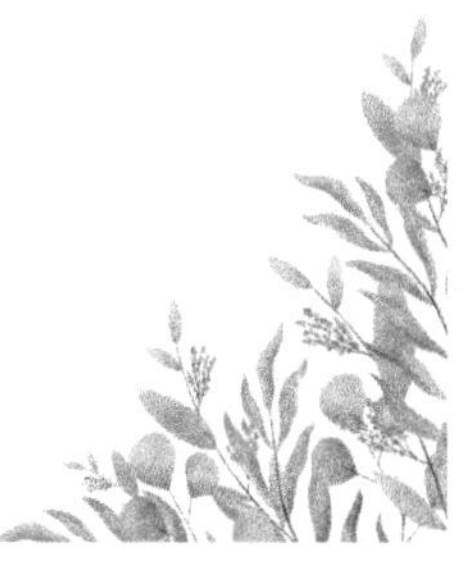

Acrest Press

Table of Contents

PCOS Most Common Questions and Answers

Most Common PCOS Questions and Answers

Q. What does PCOS stand for?Denver Pelvic Pain

A. PCOS is an abbreviation for Polycystic Ovary Syndrome.

Q. What is the cause of PCOS?

A. The specific cause of PCOS is yet unknown. Some specialists believe it is a hereditary, inherited disorder because women who have it are more likely to have a sister or mother who also has it. Most people believe that women with PCOS have a malfunction in insulin or insulin secretion that causes the condition, which is why they are more prone to develop diabetes.

Q. Who is at risk for PCOS?

A. PCOS commonly affects women once they begin menstruating or reach puberty (around the age of 11).

Q. Can PCOS damage your ability to conceive?

A. It's possible. Because it is a hormonal imbalance, it can interfere with normal ovulation and result in female infertility and subfertility.

Q. Is there a treatment for PCOS?

No, there is not. It can be treated, but not cured, with the appropriate treatment at a reproductive clinic in Denver. Weight loss may help many women with PCOS improve their symptoms.

Q. How is PCOS diagnosed?

Q. How is PCOS identified?

A. There is no single test that can definitively identify PCOS. PCOS is a clinical diagnosis, which means that it is determined based on your medical history rather than a specific blood test. PCOS is determined by three factors. Irregular menstrual periods since puberty (when not on hormones), symptoms of androgen excess (excessive hair growth, acne, or a high blood testosterone level), and PCOS revealed by ultrasound of the ovaries. To be diagnosed with PCOS, you must meet two of the three criteria listed above. The Colorado fertility clinic doctor will normally utilize a range of tests and assess factors like your weight, hair growth, menstruation history, diabetes screening test, endometrial lining, and more to determine your fertility.

Q. What medical conditions are you at risk for if you have PCOS?PCOS in Denver

A. Long-term health risks for PCOS sufferers include:

- Hypertension
- Diabetes
- Impaired glucose tolerance
- MI/CAD
- Endometrial cancer
- Hypercholesterolemia with low HDL
- Gestational diabetes
- Sleep apnea
- Depression

Women with PCOS should visit their doctor once a year to get screened for these concerns.

Q. If a woman is overweight, will losing that excess weight help her to become pregnant?

A. It may, but there is no guarantee that it will. It is possible that weight loss could help in reducing insulin resistance, which could result in ovulation or improved ovulation. This would help in conception. Losing 10% of your body weight could be enough to improve symptoms.

Q. Can IVF or ISCI help a woman with PCOS get pregnant?

A. Yes. These fertility treatments have helped many women with PCOS get pregnant and have babies. But not all women with PCOS will need IVF. Most women with PCOS will conceive with fertility pills that cost around $30 without the need of expensive IVF treatments.

Q. Is it true that pregnancy cures PCOS?

A. Unfortunately, no. However, it is quite common for a woman with PCOS to have a cessation of symptoms while she is pregnant, and many women have improvement and more normal menstrual cycles after having been pregnant.

PCOS can cause problems if you are trying to conceive, but with the right treatment from a fertility specialist with experience and expert knowledge of the condition, you have a good chance of getting pregnant.

Q. What leads to PCOS?

A. The exact cause of PCOS is presently unknown. Some experts suggest a genetic link, as women with PCOS often have family members affected. It's believed to involve insulin-related issues, increasing the likelihood of diabetes for women with PCOS.

Q. Who is susceptible to PCOS?

A. PCOS typically affects women after the onset of menstrual cycles or puberty, usually around age 11.

Q. Can PCOS impact fertility?

A. Yes, PCOS, being a hormonal imbalance, can disrupt regular ovulation, potentially causing female infertility or sub-fertility.

Q. Is there a cure for PCOS?

A. No, there isn't. PCOS can be managed with suitable treatment based on symptoms, and weight loss may help alleviate symptoms in many cases.

Q. How is PCOS diagnosed?

A. PCOS is diagnosed clinically, relying on medical history rather than a specific blood test. Meeting two out of three criteria—irregular menstrual cycles, signs of androgen excess, and PCOS-appearing ovaries on ultrasound—confirms the diagnosis.

Q. What health risks are associated with PCOS?

A. Long-term risks include hypertension, diabetes, impaired glucose tolerance, cardiovascular issues, endometrial cancer, hypercholesterolemia, gestational diabetes, sleep apnea, and depression. Regular screenings are recommended for women with PCOS.

Q. Can weight loss improve fertility in overweight women with PCOS?

A. It may help by reducing insulin resistance, potentially leading to improved ovulation and increased chances of conception. Losing 10% of body weight could make a significant difference.

Q. Can IVF or ICSI assist women with PCOS in getting pregnant?

A. Yes, these fertility treatments have proven successful for many women with PCOS, although not all may require IVF. Fertility pills are often effective without the need for more expensive treatments.

Q. Does pregnancy cure PCOS?

A. No, pregnancy doesn't cure PCOS. However, it's common for symptoms to diminish during pregnancy, and some women experience improvements in menstrual cycles post-pregnancy. With proper treatment from an experienced fertility specialist, women with PCOS can enhance their chances of conception.

Q. Can lifestyle changes contribute to managing PCOS symptoms?

A. Yes, lifestyle modifications such as a balanced diet, regular exercise, and stress management can positively impact PCOS symptoms. These changes may help regulate menstrual cycles and improve overall health.

Q. Are there specific dietary recommendations for women with PCOS?

A. Adopting an anti-inflammatory diet, rich in whole foods and low in gluten, dairy, added sugar, and unhealthy oils, is often recommended for women with PCOS. This can help minimize inflammation and support hormonal balance.

Q. How does hormonal birth control factor into PCOS treatment?

A. Hormonal birth control is commonly prescribed to regulate menstrual cycles and manage symptoms. However, it's essential to weigh the benefits and potential side effects, as going off birth control may lead to a return of symptoms.

Q. Can acupuncture be beneficial for women with PCOS?

A. Some women with PCOS find acupuncture helpful in managing symptoms such as irregular periods, hormonal imbalances, and stress. It's essential to consult with a qualified practitioner to determine if acupuncture is a suitable addition to the treatment plan.

Q. What role does a functional medicine doctor play in PCOS management?

A. A functional medicine doctor can assess the root causes of PCOS, considering factors like hormonal imbalances, gut health, and lifestyle. They may develop a personalized treatment plan, including dietary changes, supplements, and stress management techniques.

Q. How can women with PCOS navigate emotional challenges associated with the condition?

A. Coping with the emotional aspects of PCOS is crucial. Seeking support from healthcare professionals, support groups, or mental health practitioners can provide valuable resources. Adopting self-care practices, such as meditation and journaling, may also contribute to emotional well-being.

Q. Are there alternative therapies or supplements that may complement PCOS treatment?

A. Some women with PCOS explore supplements like inositol, omega-3 fatty acids, and vitex to support hormonal balance. However, it's vital to consult with a healthcare provider before incorporating supplements, as individual needs vary.

Q. Can women with PCOS pursue fertility preservation options?

A. Yes, women with PCOS interested in fertility preservation may explore options like egg freezing. Consulting with a fertility specialist can help create a personalized plan based on individual circumstances and goals.

Q. What advice do you have for women navigating the challenges of PCOS?

A. It's essential for women with PCOS to advocate for their health, work closely with healthcare professionals, and prioritize self-care. Understanding the condition, seeking support, and staying proactive in managing symptoms can contribute to a more empowered journey with PCOS.

Navigating PCOS requires a holistic approach, addressing both physical and emotional aspects. With informed choices, support, and personalized care, women with PCOS can optimize their well-being and fertility prospects.

My PCOS journey

After Paul and I tied the knot in September, we decided to take proactive steps regarding our future family plans. However, what we anticipated as a routine visit to an IVF clinic ended with a surprising diagnosis - Polycystic Ovarian Syndrome (PCOS). Here's a glimpse into my journey and the strategies I've embraced for natural healing.

Understanding PCOS:

Polycystic Ovary Syndrome is a hormonal disorder with an unknown cause, affecting approximately 1 in 10 women globally. Its symptoms range from irregular periods and fertility issues to excessive hair growth and weight gain. PCOS is often associated with a hormonal imbalance involving Androgens, Insulin, and Progesterone.

My Hormonal History:

A decade ago, I was prescribed hormonal birth control to address irregular cycles and anxiety. Fast forward to last summer when stress, weight gain, and anxiety resurfaced. Despite concerns, my OBGYN attributed it to stress and dismissed the possibility of a hormonal disorder due to my birth control use. Unsatisfied, I decided to stop birth control in August 2018. Shortly after, symptoms reminiscent of a decade ago returned, leading to my PCOS diagnosis.

My PCOS Symptoms:

- Irregular cycles, often around 70 days
- Unexplained weight gain despite a healthy lifestyle
- Persistent anxiety
- Fatigue, linked to an inactive thyroid
- New-onset acne
- Occasional headaches

Navigating Emotions:

Receiving a PCOS diagnosis brought a mix of emotions, including frustration, anger, and comparisons to others. However, understanding the root cause also brought relief. While PCOS lacks a cure, I decided against medication and committed to a natural and dietary healing approach.

Healing Naturally - My Game Plan:

- Balancing blood sugar levels to address hormonal imbalances.
- Eliminating dairy and gluten to aid gut health and reduce inflammation.
- Surrounding myself with positive influences, including my supportive husband.
- Reducing physical stress through gentler workouts like yoga.
- Making a career change to reduce overall stress levels.
- Incorporating essential vitamins and supplements.
- Seeking guidance from a functional medicine doctor and health coach.
- Embracing a nutrient-dense diet with a focus on vegetables and healthy fats.
- Exploring holistic practices like acupuncture.
- Adopting toxin-free products for both skincare and household use.

While this journey feels overwhelming at times, it empowers me to take control of my body's well-being. By sharing my experiences, I hope to connect with and support the 10 million women worldwide navigating PCOS.

Conceiving with PCOS: My Journey to a Successful First Try

Getting pregnant with PCOS can be challenging, but it's definitely possible! In this post, I share my personal experience of conceiving on the first try after being diagnosed with PCOS.

When I found out about my PCOS diagnosis in the summer of 2018, my immediate concern was whether I could have children. Knowing that PCOS can affect fertility, especially with irregular periods, I decided to take charge of my health naturally. Despite being prescribed metformin and hormonal birth control to manage symptoms, I aimed to regulate my cycle and reverse PCOS effects for a smooth conception journey with my husband.

Understanding Ovulation:

I learned that ovulation is crucial for hormonal health, and tracking it became my priority. I used apps like Flo Living and CLUE to monitor my cycle, including body temperature, fertile mucus, and more. Additionally, I employed digital ovulation tests to pinpoint my fertile window.

Steps to Boost Fertility:

To prepare my body for conception, I followed a 10-step plan:

- Quit hormonal birth control.
- Adopt an anti-inflammatory diet, focusing on whole foods.
- Work on healing the gut through a gut-friendly diet and probiotics.
- Manage blood sugar levels with mindful eating.
- Reduce stress through lifestyle changes and self-care.
- Consult a functional doctor for custom hormone labs.

- Balance the thyroid with comprehensive thyroid panel tests.
- Enhance the diet with supplements based on blood work.
- Cut out environmental toxins by opting for non-toxic products.
- Exercise moderately and avoid over-exertion.

Hidden Drivers of PCOS:

I identified potential hidden drivers of PCOS and addressed them:

- Thyroid disease
- Vitamin D deficiency
- Zinc deficiency
- Iodine deficiency
- Elevated prolactin
- Insufficient food or carb intake
- Taking Control of Fertility:

This comprehensive approach empowered me to conceive successfully. I encourage others to take it one step at a time and allow at least 100 days for the body to regulate after making lifestyle changes.

Remember, you have options, and with patience and dedication, you can navigate PCOS and achieve your fertility goals.

Celebrating the Positive Results:

After making these adjustments, I patiently waited for my body to regulate, understanding that it takes around 100 days for follicles to mature from their dormant state through ovulation. The changes I implemented gradually became habits, and I started noticing positive results.

The Joy of Conceiving:

To my delight, my husband and I conceived on our first attempt, and we eagerly anticipate welcoming our first baby in October 2019. This experience has not only brought us immense joy but also reaffirmed the effectiveness of the steps I took to enhance my fertility naturally.

I share my journey not to overwhelm but to empower those facing similar challenges. You don't have to do everything at once; take it one step at a time. This comprehensive list is a testament to what worked for me, and I hope it inspires others to explore their options, challenge medical narratives, and take control of their fertility.

Embracing Hope

It's important to note that you are not on this path alone. If you've been diagnosed with PCOS or face fertility concerns, there is hope, and there are choices beyond traditional medical interventions. This is your journey, and you have the power to shape it.

Conceiving with PCOS might pose challenges, but with determination, informed choices, and a supportive community, you can overcome them. Trust your body, stay committed to your well-being, and celebrate each positive step in your journey toward parenthood.

Crispy Chicken Salad with Honey Mustard Dressing

Honey Mustard Dressing

- ¼ cup honey
- ¼ cup mayonnaise
- ¼ cup Dijon mustard
- 1 tablespoon lemon juice or white distilled vinegar

Crispy Chicken

- 1 lb chicken tenderloins
- 2 large eggs
- ½ cup all-purpose flour
- ¼ cup Panko breadcrumbs
- 1 teaspoon garlic powder
- ½ teaspoon paprika
- 1 teaspoon salt
- ¼ teaspoon black pepper
- ⅓ cup coconut or avocado oil
- Crispy Chicken Salad
- 8 cups romaine lettuce, chopped
- 3-4 hard-boiled eggs, quartered

- 1-2 avocados, sliced or chopped
- ½ red onion, thinly sliced
- 1 cup cherry tomatoes, halved

Instructions

1. Make the dressing: Whisk all ingredients together in a small bowl and place in the fridge until ready to serve.

2. Prep the chicken: Pat the chicken tenders dry and season with salt and pepper. Create three dredging stations: one with flour, one with beaten eggs, and one with the remaining flour, breadcrumbs, and seasonings, mixed together. Place a parchment-lined baking sheet or plate nearby.

3. Dredge the chicken: Dredge each chicken tender in the flour, then the egg, then the panko mixture, coating all sides well. Arrange the coated chicken on the ready baking sheet

4. Fry the chicken: Heat oil in a large skillet over medium-high heat to 325°F. Fry half of the chicken tenders for 4 minutes per side, or until golden brown and 160°F internal temperature. Place the chicken

on a plate lined with paper towels, and repeat the process with the remaining chicken.

5. Assemble the salad: Add lettuce to a large bowl and top with eggs, avocado, red onion, tomatoes, and cheese (optional). Slice the chicken and add it to the salad.

Serve: Drizzle with dressing and enjoy!

Tips

- Use an instant-read thermometer to ensure the oil and chicken reach the correct temperatures.
- You can air fry the chicken instead of frying it.
- Store leftover salad in the fridge for up to 2 days, but remove the avocado and store the chicken separately to prevent sogginess.

Health benefits of the recipe:

This recipe is a good source of protein, healthy fats, and fiber. The chicken is a good source of lean protein, which can help you feel full and satisfied. The avocado is a good

source of healthy fats, which can help lower your risk of heart disease. The fiber in the lettuce
and tomatoes can help you feel full and regulate your digestion.

Healthy Zuppa Toscana Recipe

Ingredients:

- 1 tablespoon olive oil or avocado oil
- 1 medium yellow onion, finely diced
- 3 cloves garlic, finely minced
- 1 lb hot or regular Italian sausage, casing removed (check for sugars and preservatives)
- 2 teaspoons Italian seasoning
- 6 cups reduced-sodium chicken broth (or bone broth)
- Your 4 medium russet potatoes, diced into half-inch cubes
- 1 teaspoon kosher salt
- ½ teaspoon crushed red pepper flakes (optional)
- 4 cups kale, chopped and stems removed
- 1 cup full-fat coconut cream
- 1 tablespoon tapioca flour (optional, for thickening)

Instructions:

1. In a large pot or Dutch oven, heat the olive oil or avocado oil over medium heat. Add the diced onion and cook until softened, approximately 5 minutes. Add the minced garlic and cook for an additional minute until it becomes fragrant.

2. Add the Italian sausage to the pot and brown it, breaking it up with a spoon, for about 5 minutes. Drain any excess fat.

3. Stir in the Italian seasoning, then add the chicken broth, diced potatoes, salt, and red pepper flakes (if using). Bring the mixture to a boil, then reduce the heat and simmer for 20 minutes, or until the potatoes are tender.

4. Add the chopped kale and coconut cream to the pot. Simmer for an additional 5 minutes, allowing the kale to wilt.

5. If desired, create a slurry by whisking tapioca flour with 1 tablespoon of water. Stir the slurry into the soup and simmer for another minute until it thickens.

6. Taste and adjust seasonings as needed. Serve hot, optionally drizzling additional coconut cream and adding fresh cracked pepper to taste.

PCOS Health Benefits:

- This recipe is low in carbohydrates and gluten-free, both of which can be beneficial for managing PCOS symptoms like insulin resistance and weight gain.
- The high protein content from the sausage and coconut cream helps with satiety and managing blood sugar levels.
- The fiber in the kale and onions aids in digestion and gut health, which can be impacted by PCOS.
- The healthy fats in the olive oil and coconut cream help balance hormones and regulate inflammation.

Easy Turkey Taco Stuffed Peppers

Ingredients:

- 4 bell peppers, any color combination you like
- 1 lb ground turkey
- 1 onion, chopped
- 1 green bell pepper, chopped
- 1 red bell pepper, chopped
- 1 clove garlic, minced
- 1 teaspoon chili powder
- ½ teaspoon cumin
- ¼ teaspoon smoked paprika
- ¼ teaspoon oregano
- Salt and pepper to taste
- 1 (15 oz) can diced tomatoes, undrained
- 1 cup cooked brown rice or quinoa (optional)
- ¼ cup chopped fresh cilantro (optional)

Instructions:

1. Preheat oven to 375°F. Cut the tops off the bell peppers and remove seeds and membranes. Place the peppers open-side down in a baking dish.

2. In a large skillet, brown the ground turkey over medium heat. Drain any excess fat.

3. Add onion, green bell pepper, and red bell pepper to the skillet and cook until softened, about 5 minutes. Stir in garlic and spices, cooking for another minute until fragrant.

4. Add tomatoes and their juices to the skillet and simmer for 5 minutes. Season with salt and pepper to taste.

5. Fill each bell pepper with the turkey mixture and top with cooked rice or quinoa, if using. Sprinkle with cilantro and bake for 20-25 minutes, or until peppers are tender and filling is heated through.

PCOS Health Benefits:

This recipe is lower in fat than traditional taco fillings due to the use of lean ground turkey.

The high protein content from the turkey helps with satiety and managing blood sugar levels.

The fiber in the bell peppers and rice/quinoa aids in digestion and gut health.

The vegetables provide essential vitamins and minerals, which can be beneficial for overall health.

Grilled Hawaiian Teriyaki Burgers

These burgers burst with tropical sweetness and savory umami.

Ingredients:

- 1 lb ground beef (or turkey, for a lighter option)
- 1/2 cup teriyaki sauce
- 1/4 cup pineapple juice
- 1 tablespoon soy sauce
- 1 teaspoon grated ginger
- 1/2 teaspoon garlic powder
- Hamburger buns
- Pineapple slices
- Sliced red onion
- Lettuce leaves
- Mayonnaise (optional)

Instructions:

1. Combine teriyaki sauce, pineapple juice, soy sauce, ginger, and garlic powder in a bowl.
2. Marinate ground meat in the mixture for at least 30 minutes.

3. Preheat grill to medium-high heat.

4. Form the meat into patties and grill for 4-5 minutes per side, or until cooked through.

5. Toast hamburger buns.

6. Assemble burgers with your favorite toppings like pineapple slices, red onion, lettuce leaves, and mayonnaise.

Korean Shredded Beef Tacos

These tacos are a spicy and flavorful explosion inspired by Korean BBQ.

Ingredients:

- 1 lb chuck roast
- 1/4 cup soy sauce
- 1/4 cup brown sugar
- 2 tablespoons gochujang (Korean chili paste)
- 1 tablespoon sesame oil
- 1 tablespoon rice vinegar
- 1 clove garlic, minced
- 1 teaspoon ginger, minced
- 1/2 teaspoon Korean chili flakes (optional)
- Tortillas
- Kimchi (optional)
- Shredded carrots
- Scallions

Instructions:

1. In a slow cooker, combine soy sauce, brown sugar, gochujang, sesame oil, rice vinegar, garlic, ginger, and chili flakes (if using).

2. Add chuck roast and cook on low for 8-10 hours, or until fork-tender.

3. Shred the beef with two forks.

4. Warm tortillas and fill with shredded beef, kimchi (if using), carrots, and scallions.

Taco Stuffed Sweet Potatoes

A healthy and creative twist on tacos, these sweet potatoes are bursting with flavor.

Ingredients:

1. 2 large sweet potatoes
2. 1 lb ground beef (or turkey, for a lighter option)
3. 1/2 cup taco seasoning
4. 1 (15 oz) can black beans, drained and rinsed
5. 1/2 cup corn kernels
6. 1/4 cup chopped red onion
7. 1/4 cup chopped cilantro
8. Avocado slices (optional)
9. Lime wedges (optional)

Instructions:

1. Preheat oven to 400°F. Bake sweet potatoes for 45-50 minutes, or until tender.
2. While the sweet potatoes bake, brown ground meat in a pan. Drain any excess fat and stir in taco seasoning.

3. Add black beans, corn, red onion, and cilantro to the pan and cook for 5 minutes.

4. Cut a slit down the center of each sweet potato and carefully scoop out some of the flesh, leaving a boat-like shell.

5. Fill the sweet potatoes with the taco mixture and top with avocado slices and lime wedges, if desired.

Slow Cooker Sweet Potato Beef Stew

This hearty stew is a cozy and comforting meal perfect for a chilly day.

Ingredients:

- 1 lb beef chuck roast, cut into cubes
- 2 large sweet potatoes, peeled and chopped
- 1 onion, chopped
- 2 carrots, chopped
- 2 celery stalks, chopped
- 4 cloves garlic, minced
- 2 cups beef broth
- 1 can (14.5 oz) diced tomatoes, undrained
- 1 tablespoon tomato paste
- 1 teaspoon dried thyme
- 1/2 teaspoon dried rosemary
- Salt and pepper to taste

Instructions:

1. Combine all ingredients in a slow cooker.
2. Cook on low for 8-10 hours, or until beef is tender and vegetables are soft.

Serve hot with crusty bread.

Slow Cooker Paleo Chili

This chili is packed with protein and flavor, without any grains or legumes.

Ingredients:

- 1 lb ground beef
- 1 onion, chopped
- 2 bell peppers, chopped
- 2 cloves garlic, minced
- 1 (28 oz) can diced tomatoes
- 1 (15 oz) can diced pumpkin puree
- 1 (14.5 oz) can diced green chiles, undrained
- 1 tablespoon chili powder
- 1 teaspoon cumin
- 1/2 teaspoon smoked paprika
- 1/4 teaspoon cayenne pepper (optional)
- Salt and pepper to taste

Instructions:

1. Brown ground beef in a pan. Drain any excess fat.

2. Add all ingredients to a slow cooker and stir to combine.

3. Cook on low for 4-6 hours, or until thickened and flavors have melded.

4. Serve hot with your favorite toppings, like avocado, chopped onions, cilantro, and sour cream (if not following Paleo).

Healthy Instant Pot Mongolian Beef

- 1 lb flank steak or skirt steak, thinly sliced
- 1 tablespoon cornstarch
- 1 tablespoon soy sauce
- 1 tablespoon brown sugar
- 1 tablespoon rice vinegar
- 1 teaspoon sesame oil
- 1/2 teaspoon grated ginger
- 1/4 teaspoon garlic powder
- 1/4 teaspoon red pepper flakes (optional)
- 1/2 cup beef broth
- 1 green onion, sliced (optional)

Instructions:

1. Combine cornstarch, soy sauce, brown sugar, rice vinegar, sesame oil, ginger, garlic powder, and red pepper flakes (if using) in a bowl.
2. Add thinly sliced beef and toss to coat.
3. Pour beef and marinade into an Instant Pot. Add beef broth.
4. Cook on high pressure for 2 minutes.

5. Let the pressure release naturally for 10 minutes, then quick release any remaining pressure.

6. Serve over rice or noodles, with sliced green onions as garnish (optional).

One Pot Taco Pasta

- 1 lb ground beef (or turkey, for a lighter option)
- 1 onion, chopped
- 1 green bell pepper, chopped
- 1 (15 oz) can diced tomatoes, undrained
- 1 (14.5 oz) can black beans, drained and rinsed
- 1 (15 oz) can corn kernels, drained
- 1 (16 oz) box macaroni pasta
- 2 cups beef broth
- 1 tablespoon taco seasoning
- 1/2 teaspoon chili powder
- 1/4 teaspoon cumin
- Salt and pepper to taste
- Shredded cheese (optional)

Instructions:

1. Brown ground beef in a large pot or Dutch oven. Drain any excess fat.
2. Add onion and bell pepper and cook until softened, about 5 minutes.

3. Stir in tomatoes, black beans, corn, pasta, beef broth, taco seasoning, chili powder, cumin, salt, and pepper.

4. Bring to a boil, then reduce heat and simmer for 15-20 minutes, or until pasta is cooked through and liquid has thickened.

5. Serve hot with shredded cheese, if desired.

Slow Cooker Mexican Chicken Casserole

Ingredients:

- 1 cup light sour cream
- ½ cup chicken stock, low sodium
- 1- 14oz can diced tomatoes, with green chilies
- 2 lbs boneless, skinless chicken breasts
- ½ TB chili powder
- 1 TB cumin powder
- 2 tsp onion powder
- 2 tsp garlic powder
- 2 tsp celery Salt
- ½ tsp black pepper
- ½ tsp sea salt

Instructions:

1. Heat slow cooker on low setting. To the slow cooker, add sour cream, chicken stock, diced tomatoes with green chilies and spices. Mix until all ingredients are well combined.

2. Add the chicken breasts to the slow cooker. Cover and cook on low for 4 hours.

3. Shred the chicken using two forks in the pot.

4. Serve over rice, tortillas, or quinoa. Top with your favorite Mexican toppings like avocado, cilantro, pico de gallo, cheese, and sour cream.

One Pot Creamy Cajun Chicken Pasta

Ingredients:

- 1 tablespoon olive oil
- 1 lb boneless, skinless chicken breasts, cut into bite-sized pieces
- 1 onion, diced
- 1 bell pepper, diced
- 3 cloves garlic, minced
- 1 teaspoon dried thyme
- 1 teaspoon smoked paprika
- 1/2 teaspoon cayenne pepper (optional)
- 1 (14.5 oz) can diced tomatoes, undrained
- 1 cup chicken broth
- 1 cup heavy cream (or full-fat coconut milk for dairy-free option)
- 12 oz fettuccine pasta
- 1/2 cup chopped fresh parsley
- Salt and pepper to taste

Instructions:

1. Heat olive oil in a large pot or Dutch oven over medium heat. Add chicken and cook until browned on all sides.

2. Add onion, bell pepper, and garlic and cook until softened, about 5 minutes.

3. Stir in thyme, paprika, and cayenne pepper (if using).

4. Add tomatoes, chicken broth, and heavy cream (or coconut milk). Bring to a boil, then reduce heat and simmer for 10 minutes.

5. Add pasta and cook according to package instructions, stirring occasionally, until pasta is cooked through and creamy.

6. Stir in parsley and season with salt and pepper to taste.

7. Serve hot with your favorite toppings, such as grated Parmesan cheese, chopped fresh basil, or crusty bread.

Healthy Homemade Chicken Nuggets

Ingredients:

- 1 lb boneless, skinless chicken breasts, cut into bite-sized pieces
- 1/4 cup plain Greek yogurt
- 1 tablespoon olive oil
- 1 teaspoon dried oregano
- 1/2 teaspoon garlic powder
- 1/4 teaspoon onion powder
- 1/4 teaspoon paprika
- Pinch of salt and pepper
- 1/2 cup whole wheat breadcrumbs
- 1/4 cup almond flour (optional)
- Cooking spray

Instructions:

1. Preheat oven to 400°F (200°C). Line a baking sheet with parchment paper.

2. In a bowl, combine chicken pieces, Greek yogurt, olive oil, oregano, garlic powder, onion powder, paprika, salt, and pepper. Mix well to coat the chicken evenly.

3. In a separate bowl, combine breadcrumbs and almond flour (if using).

4. Dip each chicken piece in the breadcrumb mixture, coating all sides.

5. Place breaded chicken nuggets on the prepared baking sheet.

6. Spray the chicken nuggets with cooking spray to lightly coat them.

7. Bake for 15-20 minutes, or until golden brown and cooked through.

8. Serve with your favorite dipping sauce, such as honey mustard, yogurt ranch, or barbecue sauce.

One Pan Garlic Herb Steak and Potatoes

Ingredients:

- 2 boneless, ribeye steaks (around 1-inch thick)
- 1 tablespoon olive oil
- 1 teaspoon dried thyme
- 1/2 teaspoon dried rosemary
- 1/4 teaspoon garlic powder
- 1/4 teaspoon smoked paprika
- Salt and pepper to taste
- 1 lb baby potatoes, halved
- 1 red onion, sliced
- 2 cloves garlic, minced
- 1/4 cup chopped fresh parsley (optional)

Instructions:

1. Preheat oven to 425°F (220°C).
2. Pat the steaks dry with paper towels and season generously with salt and pepper.
3. In a small bowl, whisk together olive oil, thyme, rosemary, garlic powder, and paprika.
4. Brush the steaks with the herb oil mixture.

5. Heat a large oven-proof skillet over medium-high heat. Add the steaks and cook for 2-3 minutes per side, for medium-rare.

6. Transfer the steaks to a plate and set aside.

7. Add the potatoes, onion, and minced garlic to the same skillet. Season with salt and pepper.

8. Pour in any remaining herb oil from the plate with the steaks.

9. Toss the potatoes, onion, and garlic to coat with the oil.

10. Arrange the potatoes and onion around the pan, pushing them to the edges.

11. Place the steaks back in the skillet, on top of the potatoes.

12. Transfer the skillet to the oven and bake for 15-20 minutes, or until the potatoes are tender and the steaks are cooked to your desired doneness.

13. Garnish with chopped fresh parsley, if desired.

14. Serve immediately with your favorite sides.

Herby Garlic Steak Bites

Ingredients:

- 1 lb flank steak
- 1 tablespoon olive oil
- 1 teaspoon dried thyme
- 1/2 teaspoon dried rosemary
- 1/4 teaspoon garlic powder
- 1/4 teaspoon smoked paprika
- Salt and pepper to taste
- 1 tablespoon Worcestershire sauce (optional)
- 1 clove garlic, minced
- 1/4 cup chopped fresh parsley

Instructions:

1. Preheat oven to 400°F (200°C). Line a baking sheet with parchment paper.
2. Trim any excess fat from the flank steak. Cut the steak into bite-sized pieces.
3. In a bowl, whisk together olive oil, thyme, rosemary, garlic powder, paprika, salt, and pepper.
4. Add the steak bites to the bowl and toss to coat with the herb mixture.

5. If using, add Worcestershire sauce and toss again.

6. Spread the steak bites on the prepared baking sheet in a single layer.

7. Bake for 15-20 minutes, or until cooked through and browned.

8. While the steak bites are baking, heat a small skillet over medium heat. Add the minced garlic and cook for 30 seconds, until fragrant.

9. Remove the skillet from the heat and stir in the chopped parsley.

10. Once the steak bites are cooked, sprinkle them with the garlic-parsley mixture before serving.

11. Enjoy hot with your favorite dipping sauce or as part of a salad or appetizer platter.

Conclusion

In conclusion, the journey through PCOS is undeniably challenging, filled with uncertainties, and often emotionally taxing. However, armed with knowledge, resilience, and a proactive mindset, individuals grappling with this condition can pave a path towards healing and empowerment.

Understanding the multifaceted nature of PCOS, from its hormonal intricacies to its impact on fertility and overall health, is the first step toward effective management. Embracing a holistic approach that combines medical interventions, lifestyle adjustments, and emotional well-being strategies is paramount.

The significance of a supportive healthcare team, including fertility specialists, functional medicine practitioners, and mental health professionals, cannot be overstated. Collaborating with these experts empowers individuals to tailor a treatment plan that addresses their unique needs and aspirations.

Lifestyle modifications, encompassing dietary choices, regular exercise, and stress management, play a pivotal role in alleviating PCOS symptoms. Adopting an anti-inflammatory diet and embracing self-care practices contribute not only to physical well-being but also to emotional resilience.

Throughout the journey, women with PCOS should recognize the importance of self-advocacy. Actively participating in decision-making, seeking reliable information, and fostering open communication with healthcare providers are crucial elements of navigating the complexities of PCOS.

While there may be no outright cure for PCOS, the possibility of managing and mitigating its impact is within reach. Each woman's experience is unique, and what works for one may differ from another. The pursuit of fertility preservation options, exploration of alternative therapies, and consideration of supplements are all avenues worth exploring under the guidance of healthcare professionals.

Ultimately, the conclusion of the PCOS narrative is not defined by the condition itself but by the resilience and determination of those living with it. With the right tools, support networks, and a commitment to well-being, women with PCOS can emerge not as victims but as empowered individuals navigating their paths towards health, fertility, and a fulfilling life.

21 Strong Affirmations for Reconditioning your body

Affirmations are powerful tools that can be used to condition our minds and bodies positively. An affirmation is a positive statement or declaration that, when repeated consistently, can influence our thoughts, beliefs, and ultimately, our actions. The process of using affirmations involves consciously choosing words that reflect the reality we want to create and repeating them with intention.

When we repeat affirmations, our minds absorb these positive messages, influencing our thought patterns and beliefs. This, in turn, can impact our emotions and behavior. Affirmations act as a form of self-conditioning, helping us rewire our subconscious mind to align with our goals and desires.

For example, if someone is navigating the challenges of a health condition like PCOS, they might use affirmations to foster a positive mindset. Affirmations can be tailored to focus on aspects such as healing, resilience, and self-love. By consistently affirming statements like "I am resilient and my body is healing," individuals can condition their minds to embrace a mindset of strength and recovery.

The key to effective affirmation is repetition and belief. Regularly repeating affirmations creates a mental environment that supports the desired outcome. When affirmations are coupled with belief and visualization, they send powerful signals to the brain, activating the reticular activating system, which filters information in a way that aligns with our beliefs.

In essence, affirmations serve as a form of self-talk that conditions our bodies to align with the positive narratives we create. By incorporating affirmations into daily routines, individuals can cultivate a mindset that propels them toward their goals, whether it's physical healing, emotional well-being, or personal growth. Affirmations are a simple yet profound tool that empowers individuals to take an active role in shaping their mental and physical states.

Affirmations

1. My body is resilient, and I trust its ability to heal.

2. I am in control of my health, and I make choices that support my well-being.

3. Every day, I am taking positive steps towards managing my PCOS.

4. "I embrace my body's uniqueness and the lessons it teaches me.

5. My fertility journey is filled with hope, strength, and patience.

6. I am worthy of self-love, regardless of any health challenges.

7. I release any fear or anxiety about my PCOS, and I welcome peace into my life.

8. I honor my body by nourishing it with wholesome foods that promote balance.

9. Each day is a new opportunity for growth, healing, and self-discovery.

10. I trust the process of my healing journey and celebrate small victories along the way.

11. I am surrounded by a supportive network that understands and uplifts me.

12. My hormones are in harmony, and my body is working towards optimal health.

13. I am resilient, and I face challenges with a positive and determined mindset.

14. I am not defined by my diagnosis; I am defined by my strength and courage.

15. I radiate positivity, and it attracts healing energy into my life.

16. I release any negativity about my body and replace it with love and acceptance.

17. My body is a vessel of life, and I trust its innate ability to create and nurture.

18. I am deserving of happiness and fulfillment, regardless of my health journey.

19. I am grateful for the lessons PCOS has taught me, and I grow stronger every day.

20. I am a beacon of inspiration for others navigating their PCOS journey.

21. I am on a path to holistic well-being, and I embrace the beauty of my unique

www.ingramcontent.com/pod-product-compliance
Lightning Source LLC
Chambersburg PA
CBHW071102260726
48661CB00006B/2406